Anne Duval

Homemade Hand Sanitizer Recipes

A Complete Guide to Quickly Make Yourself a Natural Hand Sanitizer at Home, to Protect your Family from Viruses, Bacteria and Germs

Copyright © 2020 publishing.

All rights reserved.

Author: Anne Duval

No part of this publication may be reproduced, distributed or transmitted in any form or by any means, including photocopying recording or other electronic or mechanical methods or by any information storage and retrieval system without the prior written permission of the publisher, except in the case of brief quotation embodies in critical reviews and certain other non-commercial uses permitted by copyright law.

Table of Contents

Homemade Hand Sanitizer Facts & Myths 4

Rapid Sanitization and Health Care 8

Hand washing: The Key To Stopping The Spread of Infection 11

Are Hand Sanitizers Really Safe? 14

Importance of Hand Sanitization 17

3 Laws of Hand Sanitizers 24

How To Make Your Own Homemade Hand Sanitizer 27

Making Your Own Homemade Hand Sanitizer 34

Homemade Hand Sanitizer Recipes That Could Help Effectively Protect 40

How To Hands Sanitizer With Two Components 45

Hand Sanitizers That Are Alcohol-Free Are Effective 48

Hand Sanitizers and Sanitizing Wipes 51

How to Make Your Own Hand Sanitizer 54

Homemade Hand Sanitizer Facts & Myths

There are many myths and misconceptions about disinfectants. In this article, we will look at some facts to reveal myths and put them to the truth.

One of the most popular misconceptions is that disinfectants are virtually infallible and that they can prevent the spread of all contagious diseases, including the cold or flu. Although hand sanitizer can kill more than 60 percent of the influenza viruses on your side, most people contract flu from airborne agents by breathing in the bacteria.

So even if you used a disinfectant, and your hands are clean and without germs, you can still catch or spread the virus. Manual disinfection may be a stronger preventive mechanism for gastrointestinal diseases, rather than infections, such as colds or the flu.

Another myth is that they are not as effective as conventional handwashing with soap and water in removing bacteria from the hands. That's not necessarily true. Washing with soap and water works better if your hands are visibly soiled, that is if you have dirt in the hands. However, if your hands look clean, but are they mobile bacteria, then alcohol-based hand disinfection is the better option because alcohol is more effective at killing bacteria.

Another myth is that disinfectants lead to dry hands. These products contain plasticizers, which are chemicals that reduce irritation, protect, and soothe the skin. As counterintuitive as it may seem, alcohol-based sanitizer is less harsh on the skin than soap and water. A study conducted by researchers Brown University found that washing your hands with soap and water leads to skin that may look and feel quite dry. On the other hand, the disinfectant can keep your hands hydrated.

At home, you can make some effective disinfectant. While homemade variants can be cheaper, the majority of does not contain the recommended 60 percent alcohol content, which experts agree is the optimum concentration to remove the bacteria. Of course, the best results are seen with brands such as Purell or X bacteria.

However, if the product contains 60% alcohol, the generic brand will work as well as the brand of the premium store. You do not have to pay a higher price for a branded product. When compiling all the facts about the disinfection of the hands, we can say with certainty that the disinfection of alcohol-based is the most effective means to kill bacteria in our hands, but only if the product is used sparingly and responsibly.

Alcohol-based sanitizer is not only able to remove more bacteria than soap and water but is also gentler on the skin if used in moderate amounts. And when under the supervision of an adult, this product can be safe even for children. While disinfectants based on alcohol recently faced criticism, in particular, because of the high concentration of alcohol, experts say that some of these fears are unfounded. Alcohol is not absorbed into the skin to any degree to justify these concerns. Even with excessive use, the level of alcohol absorption is harmless at best. Alcohol can contribute to some dangers of disinfection, but to a large extent, not.

The Argument against alcohol content is valid only if the products are used in a way they were not intended for use. For example, alcohol-based hand sanitizer is not intended to be ingested. Still, there have been several cases where children, as well as adults, have consumed the liquid and fallen very badly. Some manufacturers have tried to address public concern about alcohol content and began to produce variants without alcohol as a safer alternative. These products rely on vegetable oils that neutralize bacteria but have not yet been as effective as alcohol-based disinfectants. If used correctly, an alcohol-based disinfectant is no more dangerous than an alcohol-free variant.

Rapid Sanitization and Health Care

There are many hand sanitizer dispensers and soap dispensers available on the market, but still, liquid Soap dispenser ensures the quality and durability of the product you get. In addition to disinfectants and high-quality soaps, there is a wide range of distributors, that this leading brand can provide. If you need it at home or in the office, it is essential to entrust disinfection to a name that you can trust.

One of the most famous disinfecting dispensers the automatic dispenser, or Touch-free sanitizer, which is a sensor made to disseminate its content once the object or hand movement is detected. Whether it's gel or foam, this seamless dispenser gives you the right amount you need. Powered by two alkaline batteries, it will provide you with quick hygiene without any hassle on the go.

There is also a desktop pump you can have on the kitchen counter or on your desk to help you kill those germs with hand sanitizers. In the bathroom, there are also pumps for secure issuance of soap for seamless handwashing with one hand. For those who are not even accustomed to wash your hands after going to the toilet can find the use of hand disinfectants more comfortable, especially those who are in a hurry.

As distributors are no more available, because of the pandemic hit us, it reduces disease-causing microorganisms in the subway and other public places is much easier and faster than washing hands. Even after using soap and water, the chances of spreading bacteria and viruses can increase, when holding the doorknobs with wet hands.

After the pandemic and several diseases caused by bacteria inside and outside the home, Disinfect the nebulizer and hand sanitizer dispensers have become more in demand, because there is a great need to have clean hands, without being interrupted by their rush to work. Some would not even consider washing their hands after using a bath or even before eating. With Purell dispensers available in several

Keeping yourself and your loved ones from illness can be possible with a proper diet and healthy hygiene. Even in our busy programs, we must protect ourselves from infection. We must also remember that it is possible to bring these bacteria home if we are not careful. It is good that hygienic dispensers are available. Keeping your health safe, disinfection dispenser should help you fight health problems and concerns more efficiently.

Hand washing: The Key To Stopping The Spread of Infection

Infection. These words cause people to run for shelter in almost any environment. From common colds and various flu bugs to much life-threatening illness, prevention is truly the key to keeping these rapidly spreading viruses at bay. But how is this achieved and what are the best methods?

While many people may imagine a germ filter masks, surgical gloves, and a full range of disinfectant products as their best choice for the prevention of the spread of infection, many overlook the most important thing... wash. Even though it may seem like a small task, hand-washing really can make all the difference in preventing the spread of infection.

Our hands encounter so many things daily, from bacteria and viruses for harmful chemicals and even fungi. It makes it very easy to infect yourself and those around us by touching. Therefore, it is necessary for individuals to carry out proper manual washing procedures before, during and after contact with possible contaminants.

What are you asking? Some of the most obvious include bodily fluids such as blood, mucus, urine, saliva, and feces. While most would argue that they sufficiently cleanse their hands after using the toilet, blowing the nose, or be in contact with the blood, there are many less obvious places that germs and infection spreading bacteria and viruses can hide.

Take, for example, a towel, a phone, a kitchen sponge or a handle. If someone or something with an infectious disease meets these items, and are not sufficiently cleaned, then even a conscientious hand washer, you can find themselves spreading these ugly contagions around. To combat this you need to regularly wash your hands throughout the day, especially when you have recently been in contact with some things that others probably used it before you.

In addition to practicing manual washing, it is also important that you perform this activity correctly. Generally, a proper and effective handwashing time is approximately 15-30 seconds. During this time, one should rub their hands together vigorously, allowing their soap of choice to lather and completely cover the surface of the hands and lower arms. If the hands are dirty, more time may be needed. It is additionally a great idea to concentrate on removing any germs from around the crevices, creases, and nail beds of the hands, how many people neglect to clean these areas sufficiently.

Are Hand Sanitizers Really Safe?

Because of the recent fears of H1N1 and other influenza viruses with many people have turned to disinfectants, to protect their homes and offices. The question is: do they work and how safe are they?

The first point that should be noted in relation to disinfectants is that they were never intended as a complete replacement for washing. If a person's hands are dirty, the hand sanitizer alone cannot penetrate all the dirt, and the fat must be cleaned properly.

Another essential point that must be emphasized is that to obtain a disinfectant advantage, and the individual must use the same discretion as he or she when washing - that is, disinfection should be thoroughly rubbed on all surfaces, on hands and allow to dry, in order to achieve maximum efficiency.

While automatic disinfectant dispensers have their advantages as they reduce cross contamination as they don't touch the unit itself, each system is only as good as its weakest link. If faucets, containers for lids and handles of the bathroom doors are not thoroughly cleaned, the result will reverse the benefits of a vending machine. The same applies to kitchen faucets and sinks, which in many cases are a more significant source of bacteria.

Similarly, the type of disinfection used in the dispenser can significantly affect its effectiveness. Before investing in a touchless dispenser, always make sure that the manufacturer recommends disinfecting at least 60% alcohol.

In addition, how well disinfectants work, it is also necessary to consider the issue of safety. While hand disinfectants usually contain ethyl or isopropyl alcohol, children may be required discretion. In some cases, children and especially young children are known to drink liquids or lick their hands after discharge. Some schools require adults to administer disinfection. However, even this will not prevent children from biting their nails and licking themselves (especially if it is applied too much or the type of disinfectant does not dry quickly enough to be monitored). Therefore, disinfection with 90% alcohol content, although more effective, entails an increased risk. Sometimes attractive packaging, disinfectant paint and smell can be a bait for trouble. For this reason, foam disinfectant formulas have the advantage of quick drying.

It is also essential to know that the disinfectant must not be used on open wounds. In addition, much imagination is not needed to see the potential danger in the storage of highly flammable products based on alcohol, in hot cars or near other sources of heat. Despite safety concerns, hand sanitizers can be a useful tool to prevent the spread of viruses, when used with due caution. Although there is no guarantee that disinfectants are effective against all types of bacteria, overall, they provide one of the best defenses against colds and influenza viruses.

Importance of Hand Sanitization

Hands, gloves or unloved are one of the main ways to spread infection or transfer microbial contamination. The use of hand sanitizers is part of a good contamination control process for employees who work in a hospital environment, or those involved in aseptic processing and inside clean rooms. Although many different types of disinfectants are available, there are differences in their effectiveness, and many do not meet the European standard for hand disinfection.

Staff working in hospitals and clean rooms they have on hand many types of microorganisms and these microorganisms can be easily transmitted from person to person or from person to critical equipment or surfaces. These microorganisms are present on the skin not multiplying (transient Flora, which may include a range of environmental microorganisms like Staphylococcus and Pseudomonas) or are multiplying microorganisms released from the skin (flora real estate, including the genera of Staphylococcus, Micrococcus and Propionibacterium). From both groups it is more difficult to remove residential flora. For critical operations, wearing gloves is a certain protection. Gloves, however, are not suitable for all activities and gloves, if they are not regularly disinfected or if they are of inappropriate design, will collect and transmit contamination.

Therefore, the disinfection of hands (as in glove and non-glove) is an important part of contamination control in hospitals to prevent cross-contamination of staff, patients, or before the start of clinical or surgical procedures, and for the aseptic preparation of medicines. Also, it is not necessary to use disinfectant on your hands before starting these applications, it is also important that the disinfectant effectively eliminate high bacteria population. Studies have shown that if, after the application of disinfectant lingers low number of microorganisms, then may develop a subpopulation that is resistant to future applications.

There are many hand sanitizers available commercially with the most commonly used types such as alcohol-based liquids or gels. As with other types of disinfectants hand disinfectants effective against a variety of microorganisms, depending on their method of activity. The most common disinfectants based on alcohol mode of action leads to the death of bacterial cells through loss of cytoplasm, denaturation of proteins and potential lysis of the cells (alcohols are one of the so-called "membrane disruptor"). The advantages of using alcohols as hand sanitizers include a relatively low cost, little odor, and rapid evaporation (limited residual activity, results in a shorter contact time). In addition, alcohol has proven detergent activity.

When choosing the attention of the pharmaceutical organization or the hospital will need to consider whether the application should be made on the human skin or hand in a glove, or both, and whether it is necessary to be sporicidal. Hand disinfectants belong to two groups: alcohol based, which are more common and not alcohol-based. These aspects affect both the costs and the safety and health of workers using hand sanitizer from many commonly available alcohol-based disinfectants may cause over drying of the skin, and some non-alcohol-based disinfectants can be irritant for the skin. Hand sanitizers with alcohol are designed to prevent irritation through have hypoallergenic properties (color and without perfume) and components that provide protection and care for the skin through a lubricating means.

Alcohols have a long times past of use as disinfectants due to the inherent antiseptic properties against bacteria and some viruses. To be effective, it is necessary to mix water with alcohol to exert the effect against microorganisms, with the most effective range falling between 60 and 95%

(most commercial hand sanitizers are 70%). The most commonly used alcohol-based disinfectants are isopropyl alcohol or some form of denatured ethanol (e.g. industrial distillates of methylate). The most common non-alcoholic disinfectants contain chlorhexidine or hexachlorophene. Additives can also be included in hand disinfectants to enhance antimicrobial properties.

Before entering the hospital ward or clean room, hands should be washed with soap and water for about twenty seconds. Manual washing removes approximately 99% of transient microorganisms (even if it does not kill them) (4). From this point, whether gloves are worn or not, should be carried out regular hygienic hand disinfection, in order to avoid any subsequent transient flora and to reduce the risk of contamination of the resident skin flora.

Hand disinfection technique is of great importance, because the effectiveness of not only alcohol, but also the techniques "rub-in".

Example:

- Dispense a small amount of hand gel on the palm of a hand by

- pushing the dosing pump

- Put your hands together and continue to massage the gel on your hands. Pay attention to the following areas:

-Nail

- Back of hands

-Wrist

- Between the cobwebs of the fingers

-Inch

Let your hands dry, this shouldn't take more than 60 seconds.

Regular application of disinfection on the hands is required, and also before carrying out critical activities. This is because alcohol is quite volatile and does not give a continuous antimicrobial effect.

Although micro-organisms are removed from a material such as latex more easily than from the skin, the regular frequency of disinfection of the hands should still be applied to the gloves.

There are very few safety apprehensions with hand sanitizers, and exposure to work is relatively low, although it can accumulate in closed spaces. Be careful when using disinfectants near open flames (which can occur when using gas burners in laboratories).

In conclusion, manual disinfection is an important procedure for staff to monitor in health and pharmaceutical areas. Manual sanitation is one of the main methods of preventing the spread of infection in hospitals and contamination in pharmaceutical operations. This required level of controller requires the use of an effective disinfectant.

3 Laws of Hand Sanitizers

Everyone should know that hand disinfection is necessary to maintain health and protect the immune system from bacteria. The centers for Disease Control (CDC) has learnt us that in addition to washing your hands thoroughly and often, use hand sanitizer to eliminate germs is highly beneficial in reducing the risk of colds and cases of influenza, among other diseases. Here are 3 Laws to look for when looking for a good hand sanitizer.

Law of effectiveness

To be viable as a disinfectant, you need a disinfectant that works. There are many products on the market, but the FDA has specially approved some substances as antimicrobials. One of these substances is ethyl alcohol. In the right amount, ethyl alcohol can be 99.9% effective against bacteria. The common amount varies between 62-70% by volume. If the disinfectant does not contain ethyl alcohol approved by the FDA, you cannot be sure whether it is effective.

Right of application

Disinfection, on the other hand, is not something that most people do regularly. The problem is that they should, but most manual sanitizers are pains to apply. You need to pull out a small bottle, break the cap, press the gel in the right amount, and try to spread it on your hands, then slide off or evaporates. It's a simple task for people with more than two hands, but for the rest of us, it's a little complicated. The best disinfectant application is via a spray bottle, which gives you the right amount to spray and is very simple to do with both hands. If you cannot easily use hand sanitizer, why should you be motivated to use it?

The law of humidity

Alcohol is a solvent that extracts natural oils from things it touches, including the skin. When the skin loses natural oils, it dries. This can be painful, and another reason why people do not want to use disinfectants. That's why the law of moisture says to get hand sanitizer with aloe or essential oils! The alcohol evaporates after rubbing around, to kill the bacteria, and then you will be left with a pleasant moisturizing solution that will keep your hands from becoming cracked and sore.

Observe these laws, and you will find a great disinfectant that will not hurt to use! Disinfection is one of the best ways to avoid getting sick, so don't worry-follow the 3 Laws of hand sanitizers and protect yourself!

How To Make Your Own Homemade Hand Sanitizer

Some commercial hand disinfection contains the ingredients as scary as the bacteria that protect you from, so why not make your manual disinfection of the ingredients that you choose? This is a great project for children and adults since the project can be expanded to discuss hygiene and disinfection. You save money, protect against bacteria, and you can adjust the smell of disinfection on your hands, so it does not smell healing.

How It Works

The active ingredient in the recipe for a hand sanitizer is alcohol, which must make up at least 60% of the product to be an effective disinfectant. The recipe requires 99% isopropyl alcohol (rubbing alcohol) or ethanol (grain alcohol, most often available at 90% - 95%). Please do not use other types of alcohol (e.g., methanol, butanol) because they are toxic. Also, if you are using a product that contains a lower alcohol percentage (e.g., 70% alcohol), then you need to increase the amount of alcohol in the recipe, or it will not be as effective.

Essential oils in hand disinfectant

In addition to adding a fragrance to hand disinfection, the essential oil you choose can also help protect you from bacteria. For example, thyme and clove oil have antimicrobial properties. If you are using antimicrobial oils, only use a drop or two, since these oils tend to be very strong and may irritate your skin. Other oils, such as lavender or chamomile, can help soothe the skin.

What You'll Need

- Equipment / Tools
- Bowl and spoon
- Funnel
- Bottle with a pump dispenser

Material

- 2/3 cup 99% rubbing alcohol (isopropyl alcohol) or ethanol
- 1/3 cup aloe vera gel
- 8 to 10 drops of essential oil, optional

Make Hand Sanitizer

Nothing could be easier! Mix the ingredients, and then use a funnel to pour them into the bottle. Screw the pump back onto the bottle, and you're ready to go.

Collect Ingredients

Make sure you have alcohol, aloe vera gel, and optional essential oils ready and measured.

Mixture Of Ingredients

Add all the ingredients to the bowl and mix thoroughly with a teaspoon.

Pour Into A Bottle.

Using a funnel carefully pour your DIY hand sanitizer into the bottle of your choice, screw on the top of the container tightly, and start to use.

Home Sanitizer for Hands with Citrus

Ingredient

2-ounce spray bottle

5 drops vitamin E oil (voluntary, this makes for soft hands!)

3 tablespoons of witch hazel with aloe vera, vodka, or 190 proof cereal alcohol (Everclear), see notes

5 drops lemon essential oil

5 drops Orange essential oil

5 drops tea tree essential oil

Distilled (or at least filtered, boiled and chilled) water

Instruction

In the spray bottle, cartel the vitamin E oil, witch hazel, vodka or grain alcohol, and essential oils. Put the sprayer firmly on and shake well for 15-20 seconds to connect.

Open the bottle and fill it with water. Replace the sprayer and shake it again for 15-20 seconds. Done!

Print and glue the label on the bottle. If you don't have the label sheets kicking around, you can also print the label on plain paper and then use clear packing tape to adhere to the label on the bottle by using tape as the lamination over the entire label.

Feel free to spray on your hands whenever you feel like they need a little deep cleaning. Rub your hands together until dry.

Notes:

Essential oil disclaimer: This recipe uses what are commonly regarded as safe, essential oils, but please keep in mind that while completely natural, all essential oils are powerful plant compounds that you and your family (including pets) can have a reaction. Never use essential oils straight or take essential oils internally (diluted or undiluted) without the guidance of a professional, and always read about possible side effects for each type of oil before you use it. Avoid the use of essential oils (thinned or undiluted) during the first trimester of pregnancy, for small children and anyone with severe allergies to plant oils are derived from. And if for yourself, your family, or your pets, you will see any reaction, immediately stop using your essential oil products and contact a doctor.

Use high-proof grain alcohol: The Use of high-proof ethanol (Everclear) in this recipe can be very drying on the hands.

Making Your Own Homemade Hand Sanitizer

Winter and flu season is in full swing, and with H1N1 all around, the adoption of certain additional measures to bacteria in the bay is never a bad thing. I'm not saying you have to bathe with your kids in hand sanitizer every few minutes. Washing hands with soap and water are still the best way to get rid of bacteria. But along the way, where you meet many germs (e.g., grocery store, gas station, public toilets), it is a good idea to kill some of those foreign invaders, if you don't have access to a sink and soap. And when you have 11-month-old babysitting in the shopping cart, which insists that so much of the basket into the mouth as possible, you will have a little piece of mind that your daughter won't burst into hives from all the germs at any time.

On the market, there are many, many disinfectants, but I found that you can make your own hand sanitizer for a fraction of the cost. Most of the products that you buy are made from the alcoholic base, but how is the green mania, more natural products made with essential oil would find its way to the market. If you choose an alcohol product, make sure that it has a concentration of alcohol of at least 60%, so it kills most harmful bacteria and viruses. Look at those labels on hand sanitizers, so you know you're doing the job and not just smearing the bacteria. Essential oils have been secondhand for thousands of years to the fight against disease, and you may already have all the oils in your home that are necessary to keep your hands sanitizer. Using essential oils with disinfectant, antiseptic, and antiviral properties will allow you to create home disinfection without alcohol. Cedar, lavender, lemon, lemongrass, myrrh, neroli, patchouli, peppermint, rose, sandalwood, the tea plant, thyme, and essential oils of ylang-ylang have antiseptic properties. Cloves, niaouli, and pine oils have disinfectant and antiseptic properties.

Tea tree oil is the strongest of these antiseptics, but should not be used by children or pregnant/lactating women. Adding more tea oil to any recipe, hand disinfection will be more effective, but the smell can be stunning. A few drops of essential oils such as basil, rosemary, rose, lavender, lemon or geranium lighten and balance the aroma.

Always pay attention to essential oils and consult an herbalist before using it, if you have any current health conditions. As already mentioned, some oils (e.g. tea tree, cedar wood, and hyssop) are not suitable for children or pregnant and lactating women. In the recipe below, you can mix oils to suit your taste, or just use one type of oil. The basic option of a mixture of oil, which is safe for families, is a combination of lavender and pine. This will create a disinfectant with a soothing effect. Add a little citrus or rosemary to increase and finish the fragrance.

Aloe vera gel is a part of all these recipes and just wanted to mention that this means pure aloe vera gel without the coloring, flavoring, and so on. It's not the same as juice. There should be "100% aloe vera gel" somewhere on the bottle. If not, it's wrong.

If you have anxiety finding some of these ingredients in your local stores, try online sources. I'd be happy to give you an uncommon pages myself.

Here are the recipes for home disinfection with and without alcohol. Mixing a batch of disinfection takes only a few minutes, but often there is a question about what you have at your disposal in the House. You probably want to do the mixing in a glass bowl (plastic may take on the aroma of essential oils, and the metal may react with the ingredients), but you can also pour the ingredients directly into the bottle if you prefer. Either way, the funnel will be useful. Add the ingredients together in a mixing container, then shake or mix to combine. Fill the mixture with a disinfectant and another small vial that you washed to leave empty. To distribute oils, it may be necessary to shake some liquid recipes before use.

Disinfectant Gel For Hands Without Alcohol

1 cup pure aloe vera gel

1-2 teaspoons of hazelnut (add to the desired consistency is achieved)

8 drops of essential oils

Disinfectant Gel Predominantly Alcohol-Free

2 cups pure aloe vera gel

2 tablespoons 90% sd40 alcohol (alcohol perfumer if you can get)

2-3 teaspoons of fragrant essential oils

Disinfection based on alcohol

1/4 cup pure aloe vera gel

1/4 cup wheat alcohol or vodka

10 drops of essential oils

It has found a way back to a more sustainable lifestyle in recent years. During this trip, she rediscovered the many home remedies and herbal recipes that our ancestors used, but that so many of us have ever said or forgotten over the years. Adding a daughter to her family about a year ago, greatly increased her desire to live more organically and to liberate her life from unnecessary and unwanted chemicals.

Homemade Hand Sanitizer Recipes That Could Help Effectively Protect

To slow the spread of virus, we were told to wash our hands more, preferably with soap and water, or otherwise with disinfectants. The resulting rush to buy hand sanitizers led to empty shelves in supermarkets and drugstores. But it did not take long for recipes for hand disinfection to appear on the internet. But do they work?

Let's look at the popular:

Combine in a bowl,

2/3 cups alcohol (99.9% isopropyl alcohol)

1/3 cup aloe vera gel

Mix. Decant in a soap bottle or pump

Shake it hard from time to time.

Aloe vera is a moisturizing cream that stops wiping the skin. This is useful because cracks in the skin can increase the risk of bacterial infection. The main active substance of this disinfectant is isopropyl alcohol (isopropanol). Most commercial hand sanitizers contain ethanol, isopropanol, n-propanol or a combination of two.

60% -80% of a mixture of alcohol by volume to kill the microorganisms, so 66% of the concentration of alcohol in the recipe looks good, if you use pure alcohol (also known as "surgical spirits"). A quick look shows, however, that is usually sold as pre-prepared working dilution between 50% and 70%, which is used directly on the surface. Mixing even a 70% solution with aloe vera, the final concentration of alcohol will be too low to be useful.

Although it is hard to get hold of, pure ethanol could be used in the recipe instead of isopropanol. Ethanol is alcohol present in spirits, and another home disinfectant that has received some attention uses vodka.

Most vodka contains about 40% alcohol-not enough for an effective disinfectant. But Balkan 176, the strongest vodka available in the UK, has a whopping 88 per cent ethanol. This could be used to make other 66% alcohol disinfection of the hands with three parts vodka to one part aloe vera. Around £ 45 for a 700ml it would have been more expensive product, but because it was sold out at all the places we looked, perhaps, that there is a market for it.

All in these formulations is mixed with distilled water or only cold boiled water. Hydrogen peroxide is used to inactivate all contaminating bacteria in the mixture, but it is not an active component of disinfection.

Glycerin is a humectant, a substance to help retain moisture, and can be replaced with any other emollient or moisturizer to help with skin care, including Aloe vera.

Compared to WHO formulation

How do these home recipes compare with who formulations? Well, it's not so bad, because both contain an alcoholic active substance and an emollient. The problem may be that 66% of the alcohol concentration is at the lower end of the actual range.

Studies have shown that higher alcohol concentrations work better and we know that 75% of isopropanol or 80% of ethanol formulations can kill other coronaviruses. Homemade products may not be strong enough to inactivate the virus as effectively as WHO formulations. On the other hand, some commercial disinfectants contain only 57% alcohol, so these domestic products would have been better than that.

In our opinion, if you want to make homemade hand sanitizer, you should go with a modified version of the first recipe, increasing the alcohol for the WHO-recommended concentration: three-quarters of a cup of isopropyl alcohol and a quarter cup of aloe vera gel. You can also replace glycerol for aloe vera gel. It is cheaper, but it will not smell so beautifully.

Always follow the safety instructions regarding the alcohol you are taking, and remember that this is only about cleaning your hands.

Do not bathe in it and do not drink!

How To Hands Sanitizer With Two Components

Sanitizers are pleasant, but they can contain toxic components. Here's how to make hand sanitizer with just two ingredients!

Triclosan is a controversial Sanitizer substance associated with disruption of the endocrine system and other health problems for humans and the environment. It is in connection with the spread of resistant bacteria, and what's even worse, is not effective against viruses, which are often the cause of colds and flu, in comparison with the bacteria in the first place. It does not apply to the vinegar of apple cider, which is antibacterial and antiviral, and quickly you learn, how you disinfect your hands with vinegar, which works and tax less.

Apple cider vinegar (or any vinegar) is as effective as bleach, which kills about 99% of the bacteria but without the toxic chemicals. It is much safer than bleach and triclosan and is usually one of the cheapest household items that you can buy.

Just use soap and water to wash hands is the most effective way to prevent the spread of bacteria; tap water is not always available, especially when we are out in the summer. It's nice to have hand sanitization during hiking, on the beach or events where you cannot be running water.

For this recipe, you can use any vinegar by hand (although you should avoid delicious vinegar). And you can also add a few drops of essential oils if the smell of vinegar offends you. Lavender is always pleasant, but the lemon also works like Mint. If you do not mind the smell of vinegar, you can use it as it is. (If you use vinegar more and more in your home and personal care regime, you will notice the least unpleasant and refreshing aroma!)

How to make hand sanitizer:

All you need is aloe vera gel and vinegar. Aloe vera gel can be found in stores with healthy foods or online, and you want to find one that is clean; no other ingredients added. It's not hard.

Material

- Apple cider vinegar
- Aloe vera gel
- Clean bottle with spray (you can buy a new or wash an old well)

Instruction

Combine aloe vinegar and apple cider vinegar in a ratio of 2: 1 (two parts of aloe and one part of vinegar). Mix the combinations well and store them in a bottle with a spray. That's it! Spraying hands and surfaces, tools, children's toys, etc.et do not be afraid of exposure to triclosan or the risk of bacteria.

Hand Sanitizers That Are Alcohol-Free Are Very Effective

Hand Sanitizers have become extremely popular and in-demand nationwide. Viruses, bacteria, and diseases have contributed significantly to the demand for hand washing options.

The spread of Swine Flu, Hooting Cough, MRSA, and other national infections has only increased the popularity of the importance of disinfecting. Public schools, hospitals, churches, malls, airports, buildings, and retail stores have all added various dispensers for individuals to clean their hands properly.

Non-Alcohol hand sanitizers have recently become much extra general than alcohol-based solutions. Studies have shown that the body can in the end become immune to alcohol-based solutions, thus eliminating the effectiveness of using the disinfectant.

Alcohol products also have a tendency to dry out the skin. They are famous for ruining caring skin layers due to their harsh substance.

Non-Alcohol based hand sanitizers are just as actual as alcohol-based. Independent studies have shown that non-alcohol sanitizers are 99.99% principal in killing easily transmitted viruses. Non-Alcohol products do not dry out your skin and are plentiful safer for children to use.

They tend to be gentler on your skin and not frustrating. The elimination of alcohol in sanitizers is attractive much more popular, with more alcohol-free options becoming available.

Offices throughout the United States have seen an enormous benefit in adding hand sanitizer devices throughout the building. This helps maintain a healthy workplace. Absenteeism can be reduced by assisting employees in fighting the germs that surround the office. Studies have shown that the workplace grips more germs due to the shared use of phones, computers, touching file cabinets, doors, and break rooms.

Installing in offices for employees is humble, a low cost, and is better for your customers.

The most popular alcohol-free sanitizers are So popular and Hy5. Eliminating alcohol in sanitizers is safer for children and improved for your skin. Alcohol hand cleaners are combustible, adding to their risk.

The CDC has recently stated the risk of alcohol in sanitizers, thus increasing the demand for a sanitizer that is free of alcohol. Hand sanitizers have many tempting benefits and will continue to grow in popularity as individuals look to wash the germs away.

Hand Sanitizers and Sanitizing Wipes

Hand sanitizers and disinfectants are of great importance in today's highly polluted environment. They act as protective masks that protect against harmful microbes that cause the disease. Regular use of these cleaners is the ideal way to maintain proper personal hygiene and sanitation. Due to the growing demand for them, the market is loaded with a wide range of such products.

Disinfectants for effective cleaning

Liberal use of detergents for manually cleaning is one of the most hygienic means ways to prevent the easy spread of bacteria. These products claim to kill 99.99% of the bacteria present on the hand surface. Ethyl alcohol present in these disinfectants is highly effective in destroying bacteria. They also come up with special ingredients to moisturize hands, leaving them delicate and fresh. Hand sanitizers are available in containers of different capacities. For example, they are in 8 oz bottles of pump, 1200 ml bottles, and so on. Popular brands that supply disinfectants include Dial, Clorox, Kimberly Clark, and Gojo.

Disinfection of napkins-convenient when moving

Washing your hands by soap and water may not be possible when you are on the move. This is where napkin disinfection comes in handy. Loading some into bags or pockets would be very helpful when traveling. Hand sanitizers are available in various preparations, including gel, foam, and liquid solutions. These are pre-moistened napkins containing a considerable amount of effective detergents. Grease, oil, or any dirt can be effectively removed with the help of disinfectant napkins.

The delicate surfaces of these napkins help in a thorough and effective cleaning. To prevent allergies in the skin, they contain lanolin, aloe skin conditioners, and mild cleansers. These disinfectant napkins, similar to the substance, usually have non-Georgian properties. Higher-strength and softness are their added features.

If you care about your hygiene and sanitation, stocking the required number of cleaners and disinfecting wipes is necessary.

How to Make Your Own Hand Sanitizer

Appropriately SCRUBBING YOUR hands is perhaps the most ideal approaches to stop the spread of germs and infections, and to guarantee you don't become ill yourself. In any case, on the off chance that you don't approach cleanser and clean water, or in case you're all over the place and not even close to a sink, you should convey hand sanitizer to secure your wellbeing.

Just like no uncertainty mindful, containers of hand sanitizer (Purell, Wet Ones, and such) sell out rapidly during general wellbeing emergencies. In any case, don't stress—making your hand sanitizer is astoundingly simple. You must be cautious you don't destroy it. Ensure that the devices you use for blending are appropriately purified; else you could defile the entire thing. Additionally, the World Health Organization prescribes, letting your mixture sit for at least 72 hours after you're finished. That way, the sanitizer can murder any microscopic organisms that may have been presented during the blending procedure.

(Note: To emphasize, nothing beats washing your hands. Hand sanitizer—even the good, expertly made stuff—ought to consistently be a final hotel.)

We have two plans for you, and connections to discover the fixings. The first is one you can make with stuff you likely as of now have in your cupboards and under the sink, so it's powerful in crisis circumstances. The following formula is progressively unpredictable yet straightforward to make if you have the chance to do some shopping and preparing time. Another note: a ton of these things is rapidly leaving stock due to appeal. There's a higher possibility of discovering them at your sedate neighborhood store. However, your first need is to remain inside.

Strength Matters

You're going to require some alcohol. As per the Centers for Disease Control and Prevention, your sanitizer blend must be, at any rate, 60 per cent alcohol to be viable. Yet, it's smarter to get route over that—focus on at least 75 per cent. A container of 99 per cent isopropyl alcohol is the best thing to utilize. Your ordinary vodka and bourbon are excessively weak and won't cut it.

The Quick (Gel) Recipe:

Isopropyl alcohol

Aloe vera gel (additionally here)

Tea tree oil (additionally here)

Blend 3 sections isopropyl alcohol to 1 section aloe vera gel. Include a couple of drops of tea tree oil to give it a lovely fragrance and to adjust your chakras.

The Better (Spray) Recipe

Isopropyl alcohol

Glycerol or glycerin (likewise here)

Hydrogen peroxide (This was the least expensive we could discover accessible on the web, however, if you wind up in a drugstore they may have stock available for less.)

Refined water (likewise here)

Shower bottle

The aloe blend takes care of business. However, aloe additionally leaves your skin annoyingly clingy. In this way, here's a formula that is not so much clingy but slightly more intense, in light of the blend suggested by the WHO.

Blend 12 liquid ounces of alcohol in with two teaspoons of glycerol. You can purchase containers of glycerol on the web, and it's a significant fixing since it shields the alcohol from drying out your hands. If you can't discover glycerol, continue with the remainder of the formula in any case and make sure to saturate your hands in the wake of applying the sanitizer.

Generally Popular

Thoughts

It's Time to Face Facts, America: Masks Work

CULTURE

Tiger King Is Cruel and Appalling—Why Are We All Watching It?

Rigging

Step by step instructions to Make Your Hand Sanitizer

SCIENCE

Blend in 1 tablespoon of hydrogen peroxide, at that point 3 liquid ounces of refined or bubbled (at that point cooled) water. (In case you're working with a lower-fixation arrangement of scouring alcohol, use far less water; recollect, at any rate, ¾ of your last blend must be alcohol.)

Burden the arrangement into splash bottles—this isn't a gel, it's a shower. You can wet a paper towel with it too and utilize that as a wipe.

If you should, you can include a sprinkle of organic oil to your mixture to make it smell decent. Don't utilize lavender. Every other person uses lavender, and your sanitizer is unrivalled.

Kind reader,

Thank you very much, I hope you enjoyed the book.

Can I ask you a big favor?

I would be grateful if you would please take a few minutes to leave me a gold star on Amazon.

Thank you again for your support.

Anne Duval

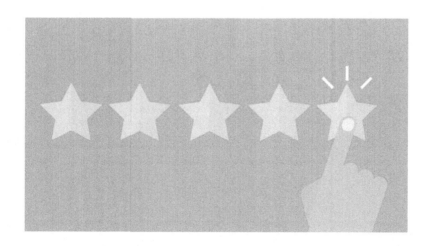

Made in the USA
Monee, IL
17 March 2022